BODY MEASUREMENTS TRACKER

THIS TRACKER BELONGS TO:

_____

I hope this journal helps you with your health and fitness goals.

BODY MEASUREMENTS TRACKER

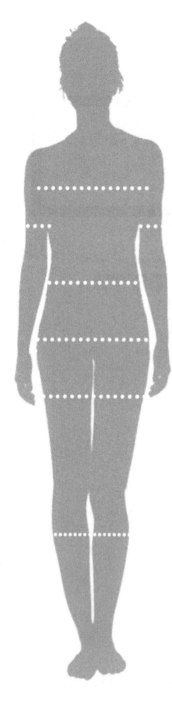

	BEFORE	AFTER
DATE	1 MAY	DATE
CHEST		CHEST
LEFT ARM		LEFT ARM
RIGHT ARM		RIGHT ARM
WAIST	38	WAIST
HIPS	39 1/2	HIPS
LEFT THIGH	24 1/2	LEFT THIGH
RIGHT THIGH	24 1/2	RIGHT THIGH
LEFT CALF		LEFT CALF
RIGHT CALF		RIGHT CALF
WEIGHT	162.3	WEIGHT
NOTES		

BODY MEASUREMENTS TRACKER

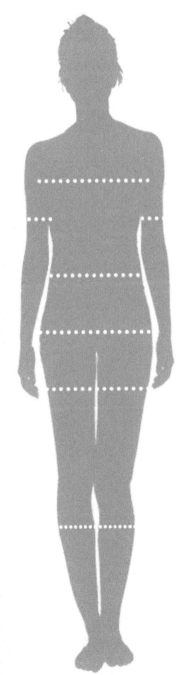

BEFORE

DATE

CHEST

LEFT ARM

RIGHT ARM

WAIST

HIPS

LEFT THIGH

RIGHT THIGH

LEFT CALF

RIGHT CALF

WEIGHT

NOTES

AFTER

DATE

CHEST

LEFT ARM

RIGHT ARM

WAIST

HIPS

LEFT THIGH

RIGHT THIGH

LEFT CALF

RIGHT CALF

WEIGHT

BODY MEASUREMENTS TRACKER

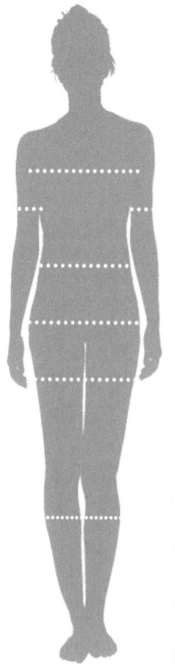

	BEFORE	AFTER
DATE		
CHEST		
LEFT ARM		
RIGHT ARM		
WAIST		
HIPS		
LEFT THIGH		
RIGHT THIGH		
LEFT CALF		
RIGHT CALF		
WEIGHT		
NOTES		

BODY MEASUREMENTS TRACKER

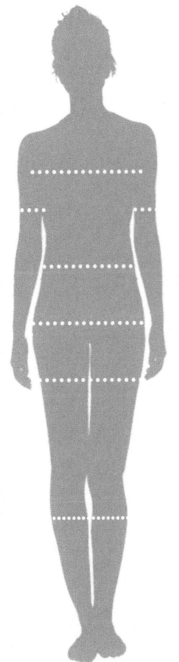

BEFORE

DATE

CHEST

LEFT ARM

RIGHT ARM

WAIST

HIPS

LEFT THIGH

RIGHT THIGH

LEFT CALF

RIGHT CALF

WEIGHT

NOTES

AFTER

DATE

CHEST

LEFT ARM

RIGHT ARM

WAIST

HIPS

LEFT THIGH

RIGHT THIGH

LEFT CALF

RIGHT CALF

WEIGHT

BODY MEASUREMENTS TRACKER

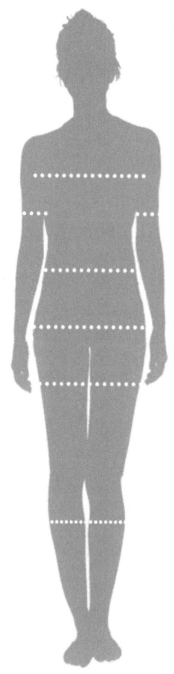

BEFORE

DATE

CHEST

LEFT ARM

RIGHT ARM

WAIST

HIPS

LEFT THIGH

RIGHT THIGH

LEFT CALF

RIGHT CALF

WEIGHT

NOTES

AFTER

DATE

CHEST

LEFT ARM

RIGHT ARM

WAIST

HIPS

LEFT THIGH

RIGHT THIGH

LEFT CALF

RIGHT CALF

WEIGHT

BODY MEASUREMENTS TRACKER

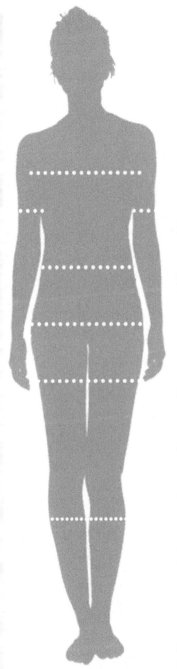

BEFORE

DATE

CHEST

LEFT ARM

RIGHT ARM

WAIST

HIPS

LEFT THIGH

RIGHT THIGH

LEFT CALF

RIGHT CALF

WEIGHT

NOTES

AFTER

DATE

CHEST

LEFT ARM

RIGHT ARM

WAIST

HIPS

LEFT THIGH

RIGHT THIGH

LEFT CALF

RIGHT CALF

WEIGHT

BODY MEASUREMENTS TRACKER

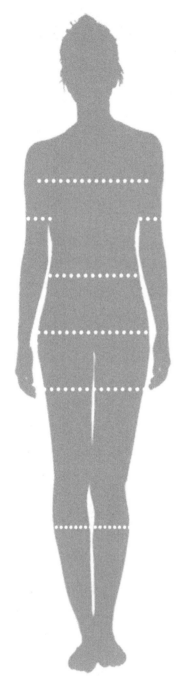

BEFORE

DATE

CHEST

LEFT ARM

RIGHT ARM

WAIST

HIPS

LEFT THIGH

RIGHT THIGH

LEFT CALF

RIGHT CALF

WEIGHT

NOTES

AFTER

DATE

CHEST

LEFT ARM

RIGHT ARM

WAIST

HIPS

LEFT THIGH

RIGHT THIGH

LEFT CALF

RIGHT CALF

WEIGHT

BODY MEASUREMENTS TRACKER

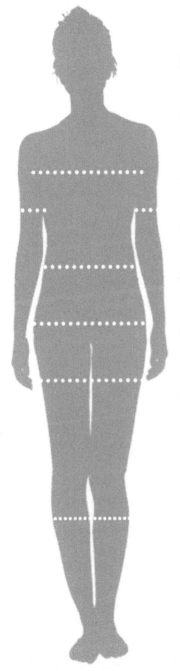

BEFORE

DATE

CHEST

LEFT ARM

RIGHT ARM

WAIST

HIPS

LEFT THIGH

RIGHT THIGH

LEFT CALF

RIGHT CALF

WEIGHT

NOTES

AFTER

DATE

CHEST

LEFT ARM

RIGHT ARM

WAIST

HIPS

LEFT THIGH

RIGHT THIGH

LEFT CALF

RIGHT CALF

WEIGHT

BODY MEASUREMENTS TRACKER

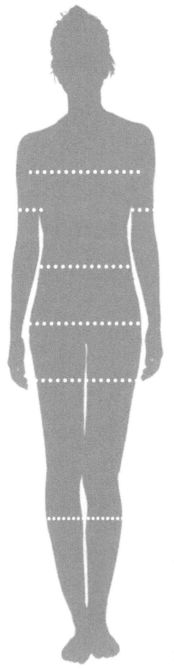

	BEFORE	AFTER
DATE		
CHEST		
LEFT ARM		
RIGHT ARM		
WAIST		
HIPS		
LEFT THIGH		
RIGHT THIGH		
LEFT CALF		
RIGHT CALF		
WEIGHT		
NOTES		

BODY MEASUREMENTS TRACKER

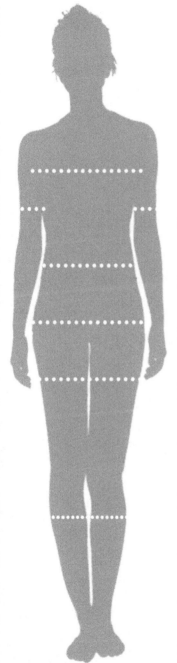

	BEFORE	AFTER
DATE		
CHEST		
LEFT ARM		
RIGHT ARM		
WAIST		
HIPS		
LEFT THIGH		
RIGHT THIGH		
LEFT CALF		
RIGHT CALF		
WEIGHT		
NOTES		

BODY MEASUREMENTS TRACKER

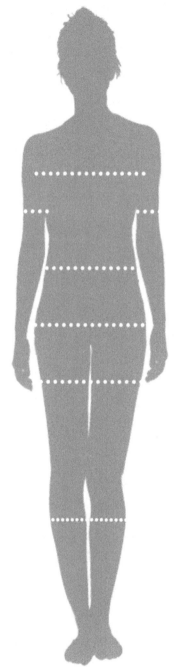

	BEFORE	AFTER
DATE		
CHEST		
LEFT ARM		
RIGHT ARM		
WAIST		
HIPS		
LEFT THIGH		
RIGHT THIGH		
LEFT CALF		
RIGHT CALF		
WEIGHT		
NOTES		

BODY MEASUREMENTS TRACKER

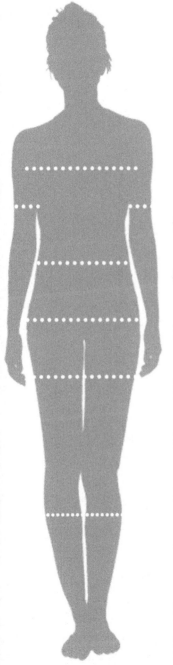

BEFORE

DATE

CHEST

LEFT ARM

RIGHT ARM

WAIST

HIPS

LEFT THIGH

RIGHT THIGH

LEFT CALF

RIGHT CALF

WEIGHT

NOTES

AFTER

DATE

CHEST

LEFT ARM

RIGHT ARM

WAIST

HIPS

LEFT THIGH

RIGHT THIGH

LEFT CALF

RIGHT CALF

WEIGHT

BODY MEASUREMENTS TRACKER

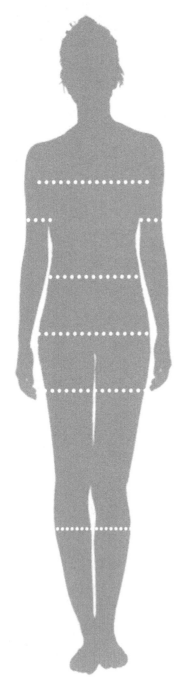

BEFORE

DATE

CHEST

LEFT ARM

RIGHT ARM

WAIST

HIPS

LEFT THIGH

RIGHT THIGH

LEFT CALF

RIGHT CALF

WEIGHT

NOTES

AFTER

DATE

CHEST

LEFT ARM

RIGHT ARM

WAIST

HIPS

LEFT THIGH

RIGHT THIGH

LEFT CALF

RIGHT CALF

WEIGHT

BODY MEASUREMENTS TRACKER

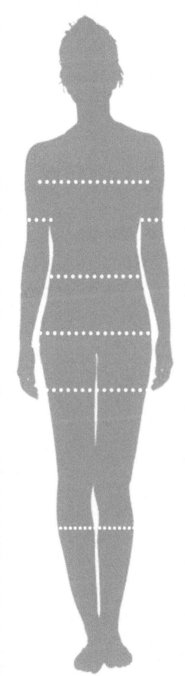

BEFORE

DATE

CHEST

LEFT ARM

RIGHT ARM

WAIST

HIPS

LEFT THIGH

RIGHT THIGH

LEFT CALF

RIGHT CALF

WEIGHT

NOTES

AFTER

DATE

CHEST

LEFT ARM

RIGHT ARM

WAIST

HIPS

LEFT THIGH

RIGHT THIGH

LEFT CALF

RIGHT CALF

WEIGHT

BODY MEASUREMENTS TRACKER

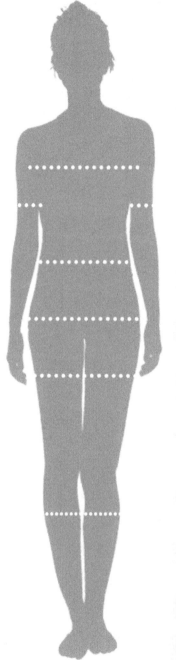

	BEFORE	AFTER
DATE		
CHEST		
LEFT ARM		
RIGHT ARM		
WAIST		
HIPS		
LEFT THIGH		
RIGHT THIGH		
LEFT CALF		
RIGHT CALF		
WEIGHT		
NOTES		

BODY MEASUREMENTS TRACKER

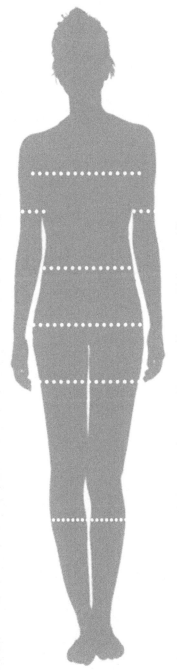

	BEFORE	AFTER
DATE		
CHEST		
LEFT ARM		
RIGHT ARM		
WAIST		
HIPS		
LEFT THIGH		
RIGHT THIGH		
LEFT CALF		
RIGHT CALF		
WEIGHT		
NOTES		

BODY MEASUREMENTS TRACKER

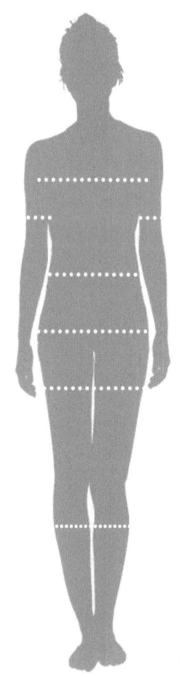

BEFORE

DATE

CHEST

LEFT ARM

RIGHT ARM

WAIST

HIPS

LEFT THIGH

RIGHT THIGH

LEFT CALF

RIGHT CALF

WEIGHT

NOTES

AFTER

DATE

CHEST

LEFT ARM

RIGHT ARM

WAIST

HIPS

LEFT THIGH

RIGHT THIGH

LEFT CALF

RIGHT CALF

WEIGHT

BODY MEASUREMENTS TRACKER

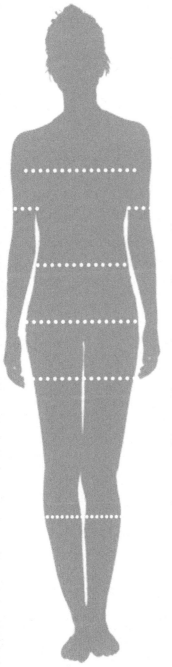

BEFORE

DATE

CHEST

LEFT ARM

RIGHT ARM

WAIST

HIPS

LEFT THIGH

RIGHT THIGH

LEFT CALF

RIGHT CALF

WEIGHT

NOTES

AFTER

DATE

CHEST

LEFT ARM

RIGHT ARM

WAIST

HIPS

LEFT THIGH

RIGHT THIGH

LEFT CALF

RIGHT CALF

WEIGHT

BODY MEASUREMENTS TRACKER

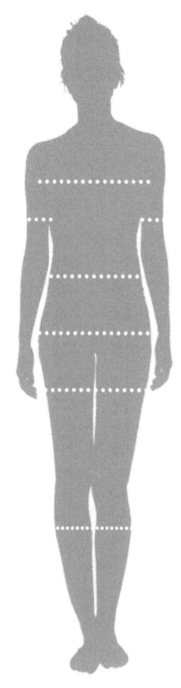

BEFORE

DATE

CHEST

LEFT ARM

RIGHT ARM

WAIST

HIPS

LEFT THIGH

RIGHT THIGH

LEFT CALF

RIGHT CALF

WEIGHT

NOTES

AFTER

DATE

CHEST

LEFT ARM

RIGHT ARM

WAIST

HIPS

LEFT THIGH

RIGHT THIGH

LEFT CALF

RIGHT CALF

WEIGHT

BODY MEASUREMENTS TRACKER

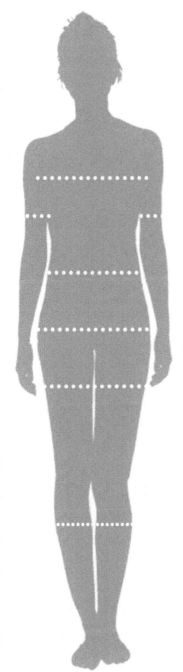

	BEFORE	AFTER
DATE		
CHEST		
LEFT ARM		
RIGHT ARM		
WAIST		
HIPS		
LEFT THIGH		
RIGHT THIGH		
LEFT CALF		
RIGHT CALF		
WEIGHT		
NOTES		

BODY MEASUREMENTS TRACKER

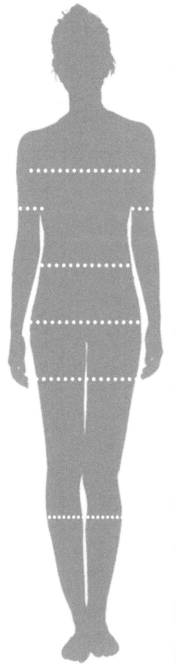

BEFORE

DATE

CHEST

LEFT ARM

RIGHT ARM

WAIST

HIPS

LEFT THIGH

RIGHT THIGH

LEFT CALF

RIGHT CALF

WEIGHT

NOTES

AFTER

DATE

CHEST

LEFT ARM

RIGHT ARM

WAIST

HIPS

LEFT THIGH

RIGHT THIGH

LEFT CALF

RIGHT CALF

WEIGHT

BODY MEASUREMENTS TRACKER

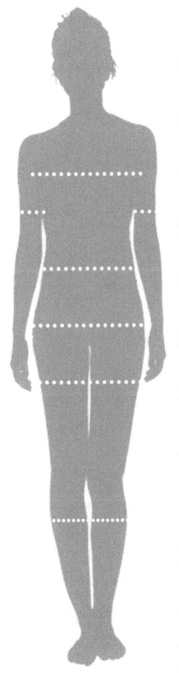

BEFORE

DATE

CHEST

LEFT ARM

RIGHT ARM

WAIST

HIPS

LEFT THIGH

RIGHT THIGH

LEFT CALF

RIGHT CALF

WEIGHT

NOTES

AFTER

DATE

CHEST

LEFT ARM

RIGHT ARM

WAIST

HIPS

LEFT THIGH

RIGHT THIGH

LEFT CALF

RIGHT CALF

WEIGHT

BODY MEASUREMENTS TRACKER

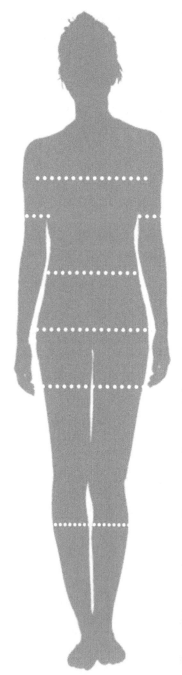

BEFORE

DATE

CHEST

LEFT ARM

RIGHT ARM

WAIST

HIPS

LEFT THIGH

RIGHT THIGH

LEFT CALF

RIGHT CALF

WEIGHT

NOTES

AFTER

DATE

CHEST

LEFT ARM

RIGHT ARM

WAIST

HIPS

LEFT THIGH

RIGHT THIGH

LEFT CALF

RIGHT CALF

WEIGHT

BODY MEASUREMENTS TRACKER

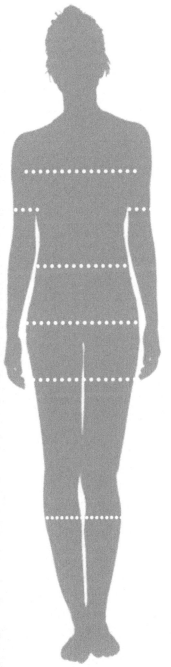

BEFORE

DATE

CHEST

LEFT ARM

RIGHT ARM

WAIST

HIPS

LEFT THIGH

RIGHT THIGH

LEFT CALF

RIGHT CALF

WEIGHT

NOTES

AFTER

DATE

CHEST

LEFT ARM

RIGHT ARM

WAIST

HIPS

LEFT THIGH

RIGHT THIGH

LEFT CALF

RIGHT CALF

WEIGHT

BODY MEASUREMENTS TRACKER

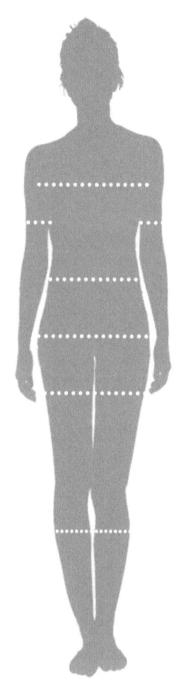

	BEFORE	AFTER
DATE		
CHEST		
LEFT ARM		
RIGHT ARM		
WAIST		
HIPS		
LEFT THIGH		
RIGHT THIGH		
LEFT CALF		
RIGHT CALF		
WEIGHT		
NOTES		

BODY MEASUREMENTS TRACKER

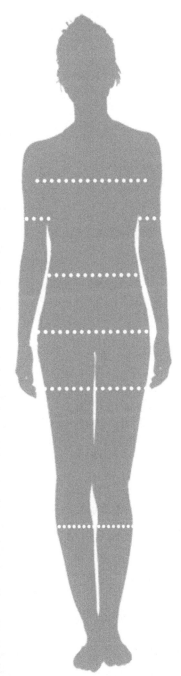

BEFORE

DATE

CHEST

LEFT ARM

RIGHT ARM

WAIST

HIPS

LEFT THIGH

RIGHT THIGH

LEFT CALF

RIGHT CALF

WEIGHT

NOTES

AFTER

DATE

CHEST

LEFT ARM

RIGHT ARM

WAIST

HIPS

LEFT THIGH

RIGHT THIGH

LEFT CALF

RIGHT CALF

WEIGHT

BODY MEASUREMENTS TRACKER

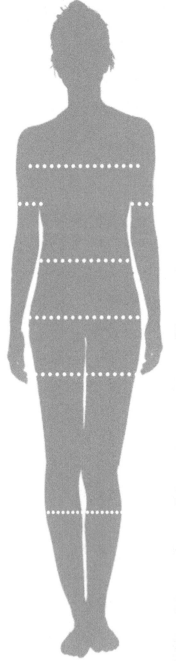

	BEFORE	AFTER
DATE		
CHEST		
LEFT ARM		
RIGHT ARM		
WAIST		
HIPS		
LEFT THIGH		
RIGHT THIGH		
LEFT CALF		
RIGHT CALF		
WEIGHT		
NOTES		

BODY MEASUREMENTS TRACKER

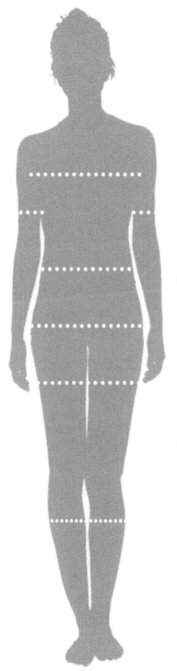

	BEFORE	AFTER
DATE		
CHEST		
LEFT ARM		
RIGHT ARM		
WAIST		
HIPS		
LEFT THIGH		
RIGHT THIGH		
LEFT CALF		
RIGHT CALF		
WEIGHT		
NOTES		

BODY MEASUREMENTS TRACKER

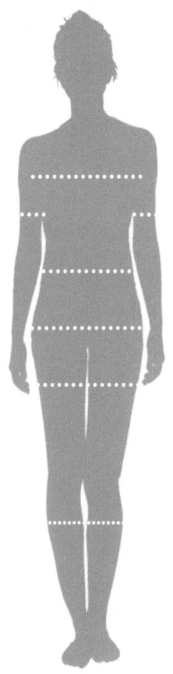

BEFORE

DATE

CHEST

LEFT ARM

RIGHT ARM

WAIST

HIPS

LEFT THIGH

RIGHT THIGH

LEFT CALF

RIGHT CALF

WEIGHT

NOTES

AFTER

DATE

CHEST

LEFT ARM

RIGHT ARM

WAIST

HIPS

LEFT THIGH

RIGHT THIGH

LEFT CALF

RIGHT CALF

WEIGHT

BODY MEASUREMENTS TRACKER

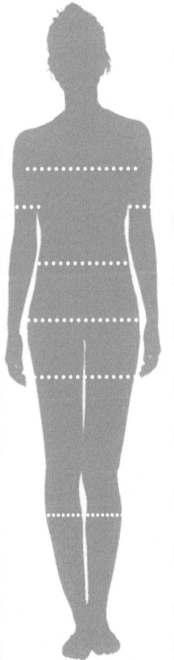

BEFORE

DATE

CHEST

LEFT ARM

RIGHT ARM

WAIST

HIPS

LEFT THIGH

RIGHT THIGH

LEFT CALF

RIGHT CALF

WEIGHT

NOTES

AFTER

DATE

CHEST

LEFT ARM

RIGHT ARM

WAIST

HIPS

LEFT THIGH

RIGHT THIGH

LEFT CALF

RIGHT CALF

WEIGHT

BODY MEASUREMENTS TRACKER

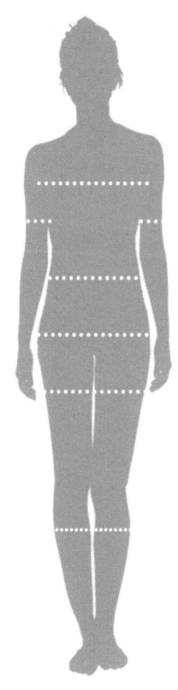

BEFORE

DATE

CHEST

LEFT ARM

RIGHT ARM

WAIST

HIPS

LEFT THIGH

RIGHT THIGH

LEFT CALF

RIGHT CALF

WEIGHT

NOTES

AFTER

DATE

CHEST

LEFT ARM

RIGHT ARM

WAIST

HIPS

LEFT THIGH

RIGHT THIGH

LEFT CALF

RIGHT CALF

WEIGHT

BODY MEASUREMENTS TRACKER

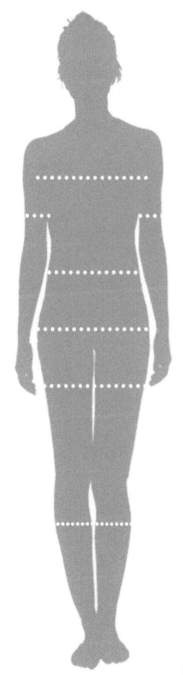

BEFORE

DATE

CHEST

LEFT ARM

RIGHT ARM

WAIST

HIPS

LEFT THIGH

RIGHT THIGH

LEFT CALF

RIGHT CALF

WEIGHT

NOTES

AFTER

DATE

CHEST

LEFT ARM

RIGHT ARM

WAIST

HIPS

LEFT THIGH

RIGHT THIGH

LEFT CALF

RIGHT CALF

WEIGHT

BODY MEASUREMENTS TRACKER

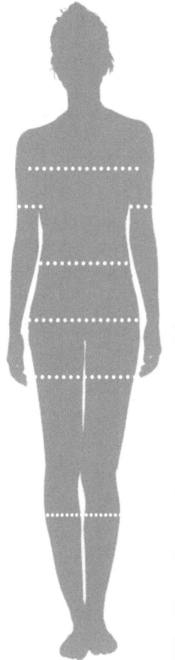

BEFORE

DATE

CHEST

LEFT ARM

RIGHT ARM

WAIST

HIPS

LEFT THIGH

RIGHT THIGH

LEFT CALF

RIGHT CALF

WEIGHT

NOTES

AFTER

DATE

CHEST

LEFT ARM

RIGHT ARM

WAIST

HIPS

LEFT THIGH

RIGHT THIGH

LEFT CALF

RIGHT CALF

WEIGHT

BODY MEASUREMENTS TRACKER

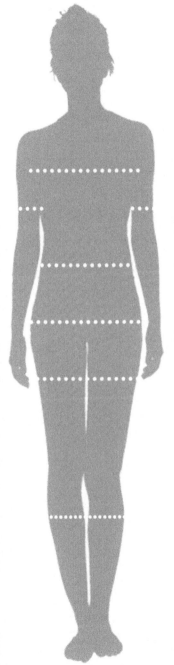

BEFORE

DATE

CHEST

LEFT ARM

RIGHT ARM

WAIST

HIPS

LEFT THIGH

RIGHT THIGH

LEFT CALF

RIGHT CALF

WEIGHT

NOTES

AFTER

DATE

CHEST

LEFT ARM

RIGHT ARM

WAIST

HIPS

LEFT THIGH

RIGHT THIGH

LEFT CALF

RIGHT CALF

WEIGHT

BODY MEASUREMENTS TRACKER

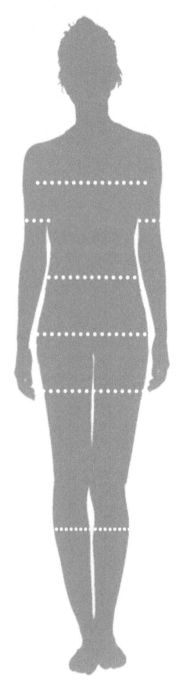

BEFORE

DATE

CHEST

LEFT ARM

RIGHT ARM

WAIST

HIPS

LEFT THIGH

RIGHT THIGH

LEFT CALF

RIGHT CALF

WEIGHT

NOTES

AFTER

DATE

CHEST

LEFT ARM

RIGHT ARM

WAIST

HIPS

LEFT THIGH

RIGHT THIGH

LEFT CALF

RIGHT CALF

WEIGHT

BODY MEASUREMENTS TRACKER

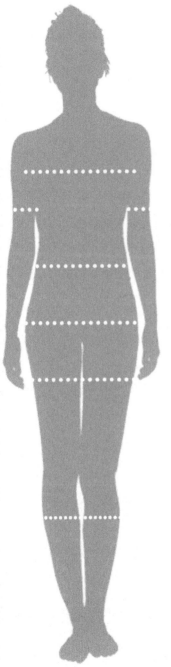

BEFORE

DATE

CHEST

LEFT ARM

RIGHT ARM

WAIST

HIPS

LEFT THIGH

RIGHT THIGH

LEFT CALF

RIGHT CALF

WEIGHT

NOTES

AFTER

DATE

CHEST

LEFT ARM

RIGHT ARM

WAIST

HIPS

LEFT THIGH

RIGHT THIGH

LEFT CALF

RIGHT CALF

WEIGHT

BODY MEASUREMENTS TRACKER

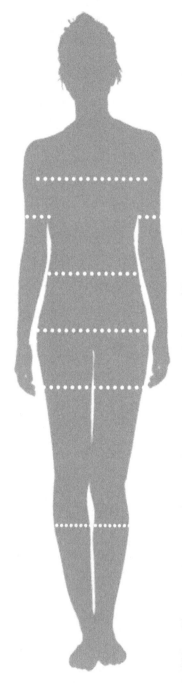

BEFORE   AFTER

BEFORE	AFTER
DATE	DATE
CHEST	CHEST
LEFT ARM	LEFT ARM
RIGHT ARM	RIGHT ARM
WAIST	WAIST
HIPS	HIPS
LEFT THIGH	LEFT THIGH
RIGHT THIGH	RIGHT THIGH
LEFT CALF	LEFT CALF
RIGHT CALF	RIGHT CALF
WEIGHT	WEIGHT
NOTES	

BODY MEASUREMENTS TRACKER

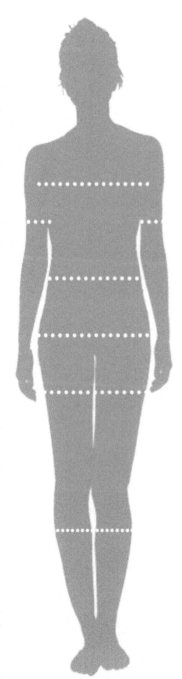

BEFORE

DATE

CHEST

LEFT ARM

RIGHT ARM

WAIST

HIPS

LEFT THIGH

RIGHT THIGH

LEFT CALF

RIGHT CALF

WEIGHT

NOTES

AFTER

DATE

CHEST

LEFT ARM

RIGHT ARM

WAIST

HIPS

LEFT THIGH

RIGHT THIGH

LEFT CALF

RIGHT CALF

WEIGHT

BODY MEASUREMENTS TRACKER

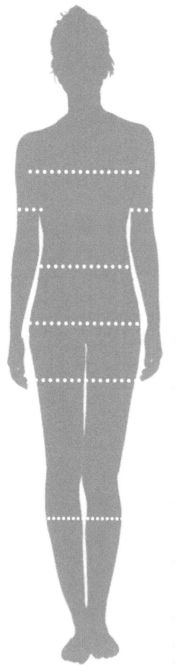

	BEFORE	AFTER
DATE		
CHEST		
LEFT ARM		
RIGHT ARM		
WAIST		
HIPS		
LEFT THIGH		
RIGHT THIGH		
LEFT CALF		
RIGHT CALF		
WEIGHT		
NOTES		

BODY MEASUREMENTS TRACKER

BEFORE

AFTER

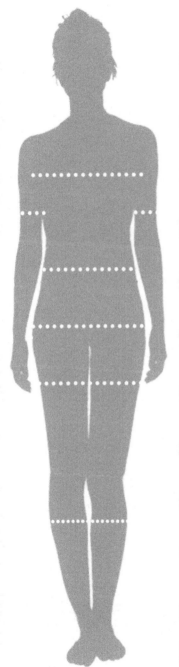

BEFORE	AFTER
DATE	DATE
CHEST	CHEST
LEFT ARM	LEFT ARM
RIGHT ARM	RIGHT ARM
WAIST	WAIST
HIPS	HIPS
LEFT THIGH	LEFT THIGH
RIGHT THIGH	RIGHT THIGH
LEFT CALF	LEFT CALF
RIGHT CALF	RIGHT CALF
WEIGHT	WEIGHT
NOTES	

BODY MEASUREMENTS TRACKER

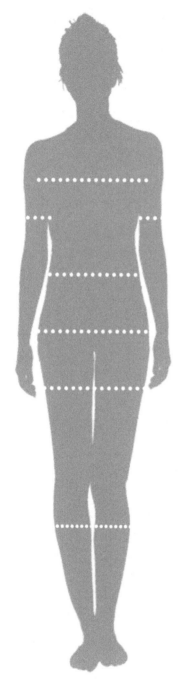

	BEFORE	AFTER
DATE		DATE
CHEST		CHEST
LEFT ARM		LEFT ARM
RIGHT ARM		RIGHT ARM
WAIST		WAIST
HIPS		HIPS
LEFT THIGH		LEFT THIGH
RIGHT THIGH		RIGHT THIGH
LEFT CALF		LEFT CALF
RIGHT CALF		RIGHT CALF
WEIGHT		WEIGHT
NOTES		

BODY MEASUREMENTS TRACKER

BEFORE

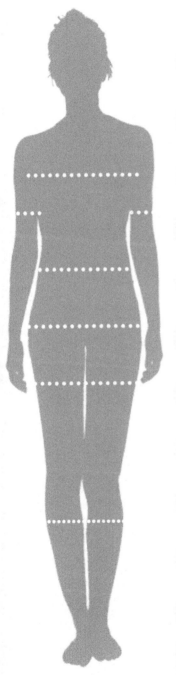

DATE

CHEST

LEFT ARM

RIGHT ARM

WAIST

HIPS

LEFT THIGH

RIGHT THIGH

LEFT CALF

RIGHT CALF

WEIGHT

NOTES

AFTER

DATE

CHEST

LEFT ARM

RIGHT ARM

WAIST

HIPS

LEFT THIGH

RIGHT THIGH

LEFT CALF

RIGHT CALF

WEIGHT

BODY MEASUREMENTS TRACKER

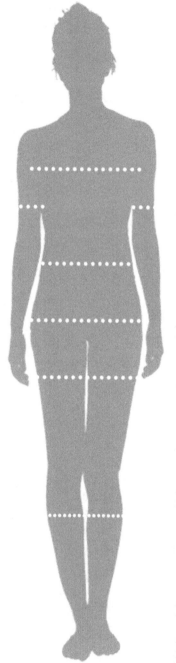

BEFORE

DATE

CHEST

LEFT ARM

RIGHT ARM

WAIST

HIPS

LEFT THIGH

RIGHT THIGH

LEFT CALF

RIGHT CALF

WEIGHT

NOTES

AFTER

DATE

CHEST

LEFT ARM

RIGHT ARM

WAIST

HIPS

LEFT THIGH

RIGHT THIGH

LEFT CALF

RIGHT CALF

WEIGHT

BODY MEASUREMENTS TRACKER

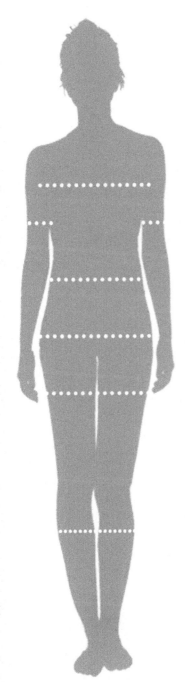

BEFORE

DATE

CHEST

LEFT ARM

RIGHT ARM

WAIST

HIPS

LEFT THIGH

RIGHT THIGH

LEFT CALF

RIGHT CALF

WEIGHT

NOTES

AFTER

DATE

CHEST

LEFT ARM

RIGHT ARM

WAIST

HIPS

LEFT THIGH

RIGHT THIGH

LEFT CALF

RIGHT CALF

WEIGHT

BODY MEASUREMENTS TRACKER

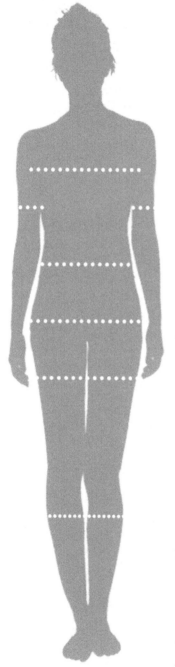

	BEFORE	AFTER
DATE		
CHEST		
LEFT ARM		
RIGHT ARM		
WAIST		
HIPS		
LEFT THIGH		
RIGHT THIGH		
LEFT CALF		
RIGHT CALF		
WEIGHT		
NOTES		

BODY MEASUREMENTS TRACKER

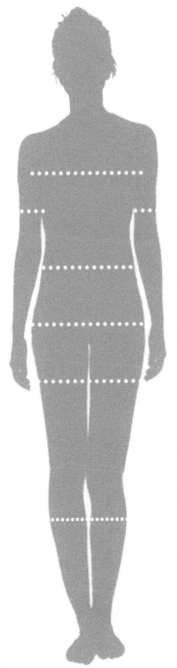

BEFORE

DATE

CHEST

LEFT ARM

RIGHT ARM

WAIST

HIPS

LEFT THIGH

RIGHT THIGH

LEFT CALF

RIGHT CALF

WEIGHT

NOTES

AFTER

DATE

CHEST

LEFT ARM

RIGHT ARM

WAIST

HIPS

LEFT THIGH

RIGHT THIGH

LEFT CALF

RIGHT CALF

WEIGHT

BODY MEASUREMENTS TRACKER

BEFORE   AFTER

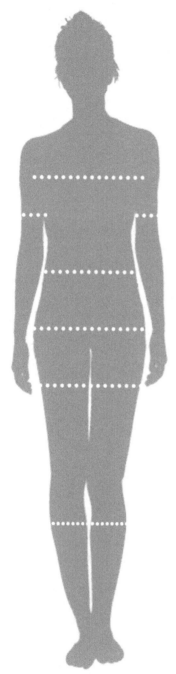

BEFORE	AFTER
DATE	DATE
CHEST	CHEST
LEFT ARM	LEFT ARM
RIGHT ARM	RIGHT ARM
WAIST	WAIST
HIPS	HIPS
LEFT THIGH	LEFT THIGH
RIGHT THIGH	RIGHT THIGH
LEFT CALF	LEFT CALF
RIGHT CALF	RIGHT CALF
WEIGHT	WEIGHT
NOTES	

BODY MEASUREMENTS TRACKER

BEFORE

AFTER

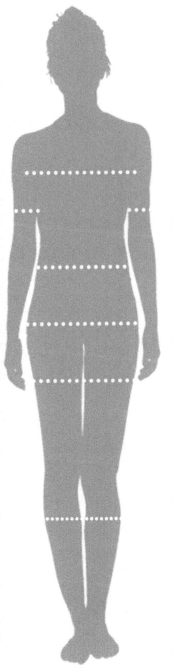

BEFORE	AFTER
DATE	DATE
CHEST	CHEST
LEFT ARM	LEFT ARM
RIGHT ARM	RIGHT ARM
WAIST	WAIST
HIPS	HIPS
LEFT THIGH	LEFT THIGH
RIGHT THIGH	RIGHT THIGH
LEFT CALF	LEFT CALF
RIGHT CALF	RIGHT CALF
WEIGHT	WEIGHT
NOTES	

BODY MEASUREMENTS TRACKER

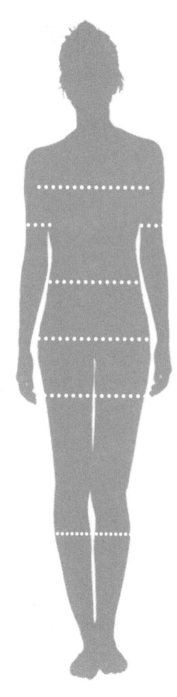

BEFORE	AFTER
DATE	DATE
CHEST	CHEST
LEFT ARM	LEFT ARM
RIGHT ARM	RIGHT ARM
WAIST	WAIST
HIPS	HIPS
LEFT THIGH	LEFT THIGH
RIGHT THIGH	RIGHT THIGH
LEFT CALF	LEFT CALF
RIGHT CALF	RIGHT CALF
WEIGHT	WEIGHT
NOTES	

BODY MEASUREMENTS TRACKER

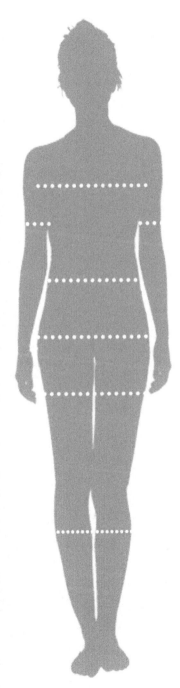

BEFORE

DATE

CHEST

LEFT ARM

RIGHT ARM

WAIST

HIPS

LEFT THIGH

RIGHT THIGH

LEFT CALF

RIGHT CALF

WEIGHT

NOTES

AFTER

DATE

CHEST

LEFT ARM

RIGHT ARM

WAIST

HIPS

LEFT THIGH

RIGHT THIGH

LEFT CALF

RIGHT CALF

WEIGHT

BODY MEASUREMENTS TRACKER

BEFORE

AFTER

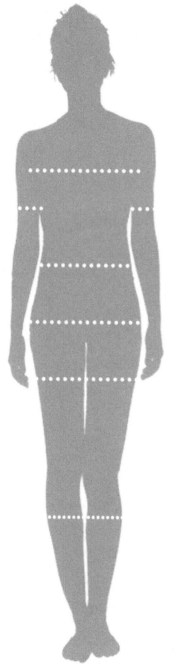

BEFORE	AFTER
DATE	DATE
CHEST	CHEST
LEFT ARM	LEFT ARM
RIGHT ARM	RIGHT ARM
WAIST	WAIST
HIPS	HIPS
LEFT THIGH	LEFT THIGH
RIGHT THIGH	RIGHT THIGH
LEFT CALF	LEFT CALF
RIGHT CALF	RIGHT CALF
WEIGHT	WEIGHT
NOTES	

BODY MEASUREMENTS TRACKER

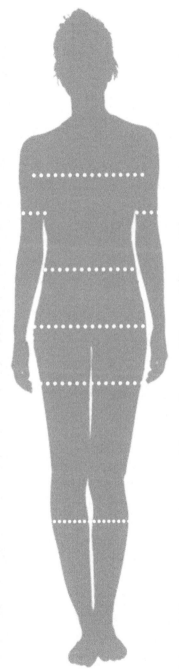

	BEFORE	AFTER
DATE		
CHEST		
LEFT ARM		
RIGHT ARM		
WAIST		
HIPS		
LEFT THIGH		
RIGHT THIGH		
LEFT CALF		
RIGHT CALF		
WEIGHT		
NOTES		

BODY MEASUREMENTS TRACKER

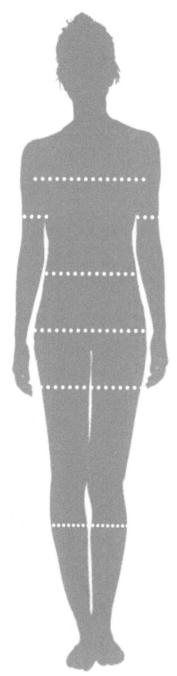

BEFORE

DATE

CHEST

LEFT ARM

RIGHT ARM

WAIST

HIPS

LEFT THIGH

RIGHT THIGH

LEFT CALF

RIGHT CALF

WEIGHT

NOTES

AFTER

DATE

CHEST

LEFT ARM

RIGHT ARM

WAIST

HIPS

LEFT THIGH

RIGHT THIGH

LEFT CALF

RIGHT CALF

WEIGHT

BODY MEASUREMENTS TRACKER

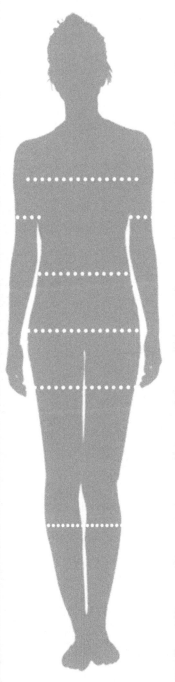

BEFORE	AFTER
DATE	DATE
CHEST	CHEST
LEFT ARM	LEFT ARM
RIGHT ARM	RIGHT ARM
WAIST	WAIST
HIPS	HIPS
LEFT THIGH	LEFT THIGH
RIGHT THIGH	RIGHT THIGH
LEFT CALF	LEFT CALF
RIGHT CALF	RIGHT CALF
WEIGHT	WEIGHT
NOTES	

BODY MEASUREMENTS TRACKER

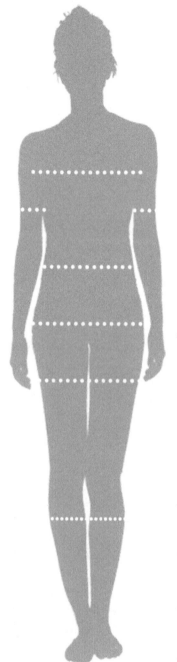

BEFORE

DATE

CHEST

LEFT ARM

RIGHT ARM

WAIST

HIPS

LEFT THIGH

RIGHT THIGH

LEFT CALF

RIGHT CALF

WEIGHT

NOTES

AFTER

DATE

CHEST

LEFT ARM

RIGHT ARM

WAIST

HIPS

LEFT THIGH

RIGHT THIGH

LEFT CALF

RIGHT CALF

WEIGHT

BODY MEASUREMENTS TRACKER

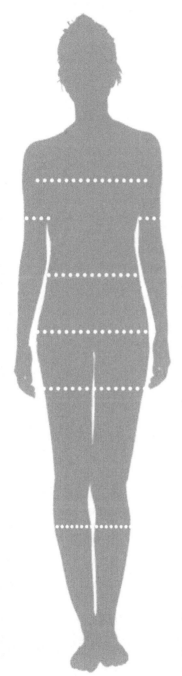

BEFORE

DATE

CHEST

LEFT ARM

RIGHT ARM

WAIST

HIPS

LEFT THIGH

RIGHT THIGH

LEFT CALF

RIGHT CALF

WEIGHT

NOTES

AFTER

DATE

CHEST

LEFT ARM

RIGHT ARM

WAIST

HIPS

LEFT THIGH

RIGHT THIGH

LEFT CALF

RIGHT CALF

WEIGHT

BODY MEASUREMENTS TRACKER

BEFORE

AFTER

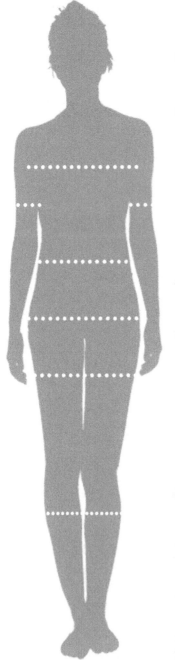

BEFORE	AFTER
DATE	DATE
CHEST	CHEST
LEFT ARM	LEFT ARM
RIGHT ARM	RIGHT ARM
WAIST	WAIST
HIPS	HIPS
LEFT THIGH	LEFT THIGH
RIGHT THIGH	RIGHT THIGH
LEFT CALF	LEFT CALF
RIGHT CALF	RIGHT CALF
WEIGHT	WEIGHT
NOTES	

BODY MEASUREMENTS TRACKER

BEFORE

AFTER

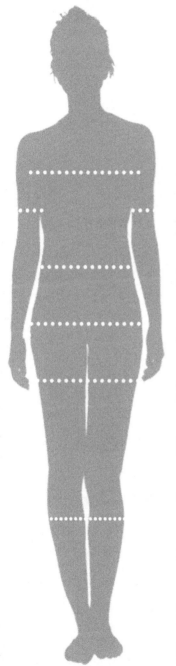

BEFORE	AFTER
DATE	DATE
CHEST	CHEST
LEFT ARM	LEFT ARM
RIGHT ARM	RIGHT ARM
WAIST	WAIST
HIPS	HIPS
LEFT THIGH	LEFT THIGH
RIGHT THIGH	RIGHT THIGH
LEFT CALF	LEFT CALF
RIGHT CALF	RIGHT CALF
WEIGHT	WEIGHT
NOTES	

BODY MEASUREMENTS TRACKER

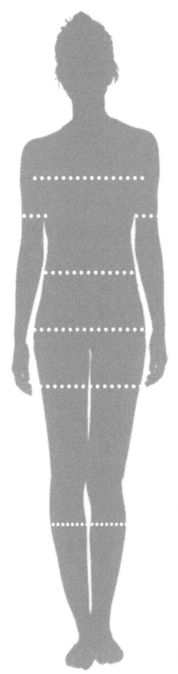

BEFORE

DATE

CHEST

LEFT ARM

RIGHT ARM

WAIST

HIPS

LEFT THIGH

RIGHT THIGH

LEFT CALF

RIGHT CALF

WEIGHT

NOTES

AFTER

DATE

CHEST

LEFT ARM

RIGHT ARM

WAIST

HIPS

LEFT THIGH

RIGHT THIGH

LEFT CALF

RIGHT CALF

WEIGHT

BODY MEASUREMENTS TRACKER

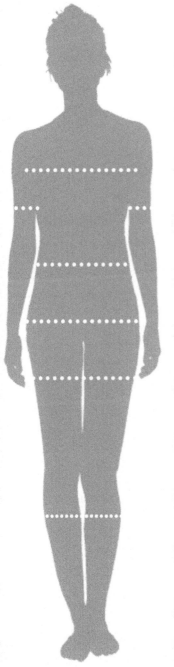

BEFORE

DATE

CHEST

LEFT ARM

RIGHT ARM

WAIST

HIPS

LEFT THIGH

RIGHT THIGH

LEFT CALF

RIGHT CALF

WEIGHT

NOTES

AFTER

DATE

CHEST

LEFT ARM

RIGHT ARM

WAIST

HIPS

LEFT THIGH

RIGHT THIGH

LEFT CALF

RIGHT CALF

WEIGHT

BODY MEASUREMENTS TRACKER

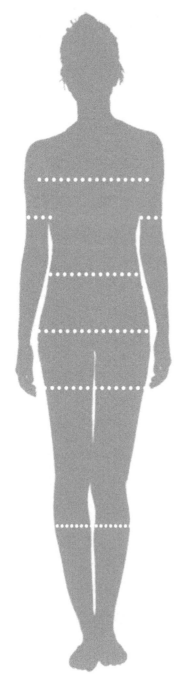

	BEFORE	AFTER
DATE		
CHEST		
LEFT ARM		
RIGHT ARM		
WAIST		
HIPS		
LEFT THIGH		
RIGHT THIGH		
LEFT CALF		
RIGHT CALF		
WEIGHT		
NOTES		

BODY MEASUREMENTS TRACKER

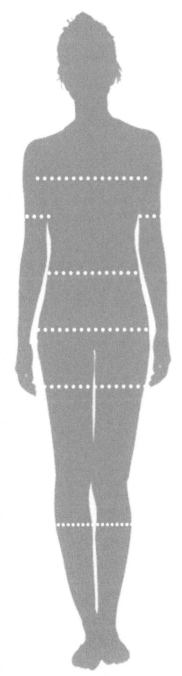

	BEFORE	AFTER
DATE		
CHEST		
LEFT ARM		
RIGHT ARM		
WAIST		
HIPS		
LEFT THIGH		
RIGHT THIGH		
LEFT CALF		
RIGHT CALF		
WEIGHT		
NOTES		

BODY MEASUREMENTS TRACKER

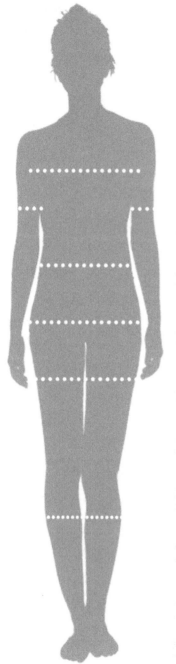

	BEFORE	AFTER
DATE		
CHEST		
LEFT ARM		
RIGHT ARM		
WAIST		
HIPS		
LEFT THIGH		
RIGHT THIGH		
LEFT CALF		
RIGHT CALF		
WEIGHT		
NOTES		

BODY MEASUREMENTS TRACKER

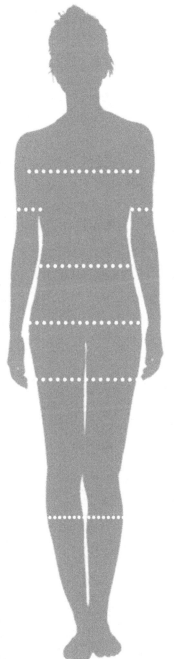

BEFORE

DATE

CHEST

LEFT ARM

RIGHT ARM

WAIST

HIPS

LEFT THIGH

RIGHT THIGH

LEFT CALF

RIGHT CALF

WEIGHT

NOTES

AFTER

DATE

CHEST

LEFT ARM

RIGHT ARM

WAIST

HIPS

LEFT THIGH

RIGHT THIGH

LEFT CALF

RIGHT CALF

WEIGHT

BODY MEASUREMENTS TRACKER

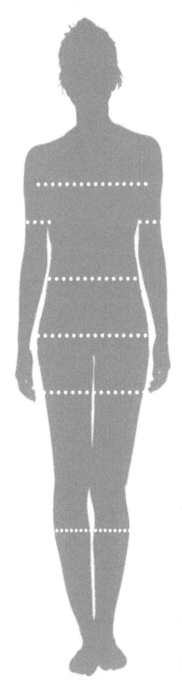

BEFORE

DATE

CHEST

LEFT ARM

RIGHT ARM

WAIST

HIPS

LEFT THIGH

RIGHT THIGH

LEFT CALF

RIGHT CALF

WEIGHT

NOTES

AFTER

DATE

CHEST

LEFT ARM

RIGHT ARM

WAIST

HIPS

LEFT THIGH

RIGHT THIGH

LEFT CALF

RIGHT CALF

WEIGHT

BODY MEASUREMENTS TRACKER

BEFORE

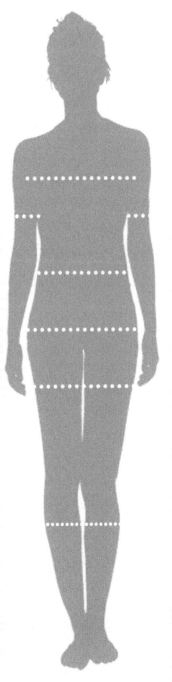

DATE

CHEST

LEFT ARM

RIGHT ARM

WAIST

HIPS

LEFT THIGH

RIGHT THIGH

LEFT CALF

RIGHT CALF

WEIGHT

NOTES

AFTER

DATE

CHEST

LEFT ARM

RIGHT ARM

WAIST

HIPS

LEFT THIGH

RIGHT THIGH

LEFT CALF

RIGHT CALF

WEIGHT

BODY MEASUREMENTS TRACKER

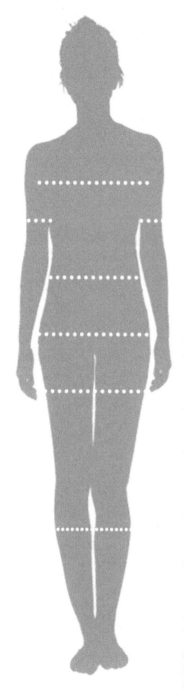

BEFORE

DATE

CHEST

LEFT ARM

RIGHT ARM

WAIST

HIPS

LEFT THIGH

RIGHT THIGH

LEFT CALF

RIGHT CALF

WEIGHT

NOTES

AFTER

DATE

CHEST

LEFT ARM

RIGHT ARM

WAIST

HIPS

LEFT THIGH

RIGHT THIGH

LEFT CALF

RIGHT CALF

WEIGHT

BODY MEASUREMENTS TRACKER

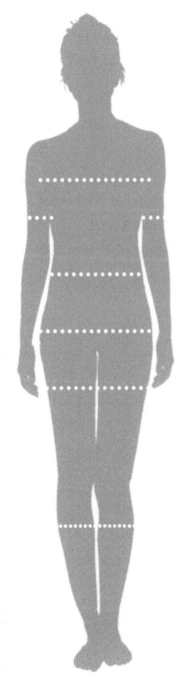

BEFORE

DATE

CHEST

LEFT ARM

RIGHT ARM

WAIST

HIPS

LEFT THIGH

RIGHT THIGH

LEFT CALF

RIGHT CALF

WEIGHT

NOTES

AFTER

DATE

CHEST

LEFT ARM

RIGHT ARM

WAIST

HIPS

LEFT THIGH

RIGHT THIGH

LEFT CALF

RIGHT CALF

WEIGHT

BODY MEASUREMENTS TRACKER

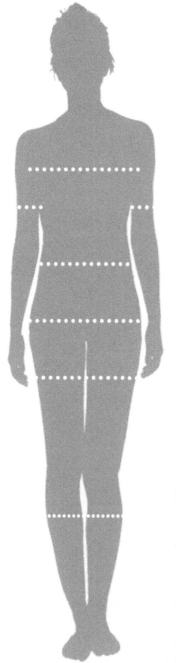

BEFORE

DATE

CHEST

LEFT ARM

RIGHT ARM

WAIST

HIPS

LEFT THIGH

RIGHT THIGH

LEFT CALF

RIGHT CALF

WEIGHT

NOTES

AFTER

DATE

CHEST

LEFT ARM

RIGHT ARM

WAIST

HIPS

LEFT THIGH

RIGHT THIGH

LEFT CALF

RIGHT CALF

WEIGHT

BODY MEASUREMENTS TRACKER

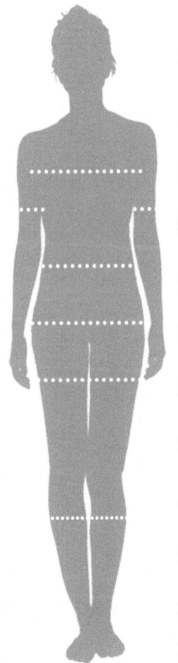

	BEFORE	AFTER
DATE		
CHEST		
LEFT ARM		
RIGHT ARM		
WAIST		
HIPS		
LEFT THIGH		
RIGHT THIGH		
LEFT CALF		
RIGHT CALF		
WEIGHT		
NOTES		

BODY MEASUREMENTS TRACKER

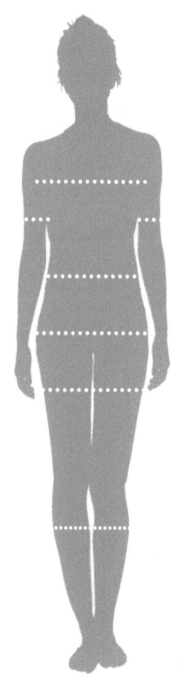

BEFORE

DATE

CHEST

LEFT ARM

RIGHT ARM

WAIST

HIPS

LEFT THIGH

RIGHT THIGH

LEFT CALF

RIGHT CALF

WEIGHT

NOTES

AFTER

DATE

CHEST

LEFT ARM

RIGHT ARM

WAIST

HIPS

LEFT THIGH

RIGHT THIGH

LEFT CALF

RIGHT CALF

WEIGHT

BODY MEASUREMENTS TRACKER

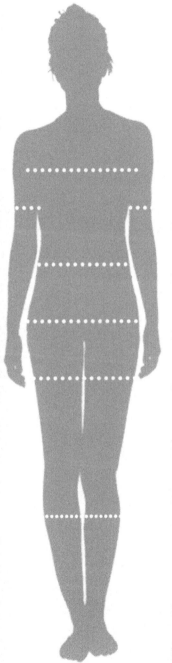

BEFORE

DATE

CHEST

LEFT ARM

RIGHT ARM

WAIST

HIPS

LEFT THIGH

RIGHT THIGH

LEFT CALF

RIGHT CALF

WEIGHT

NOTES

AFTER

DATE

CHEST

LEFT ARM

RIGHT ARM

WAIST

HIPS

LEFT THIGH

RIGHT THIGH

LEFT CALF

RIGHT CALF

WEIGHT

BODY MEASUREMENTS TRACKER

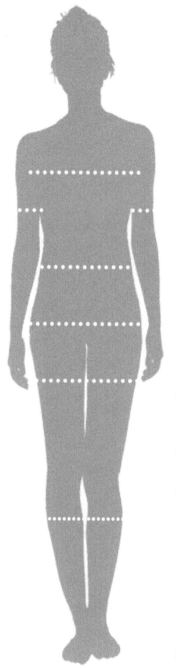

BEFORE

DATE

CHEST

LEFT ARM

RIGHT ARM

WAIST

HIPS

LEFT THIGH

RIGHT THIGH

LEFT CALF

RIGHT CALF

WEIGHT

NOTES

AFTER

DATE

CHEST

LEFT ARM

RIGHT ARM

WAIST

HIPS

LEFT THIGH

RIGHT THIGH

LEFT CALF

RIGHT CALF

WEIGHT

BODY MEASUREMENTS TRACKER

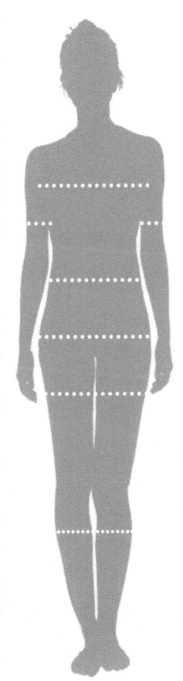

BEFORE

DATE

CHEST

LEFT ARM

RIGHT ARM

WAIST

HIPS

LEFT THIGH

RIGHT THIGH

LEFT CALF

RIGHT CALF

WEIGHT

NOTES

AFTER

DATE

CHEST

LEFT ARM

RIGHT ARM

WAIST

HIPS

LEFT THIGH

RIGHT THIGH

LEFT CALF

RIGHT CALF

WEIGHT

BODY MEASUREMENTS TRACKER

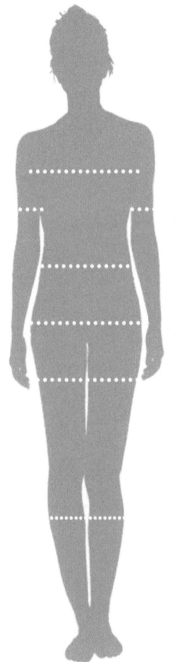

	BEFORE	AFTER
DATE		
CHEST		
LEFT ARM		
RIGHT ARM		
WAIST		
HIPS		
LEFT THIGH		
RIGHT THIGH		
LEFT CALF		
RIGHT CALF		
WEIGHT		
NOTES		

BODY MEASUREMENTS TRACKER

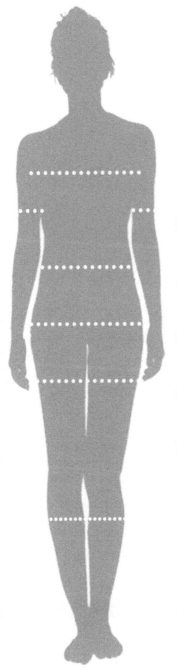

BEFORE

DATE

CHEST

LEFT ARM

RIGHT ARM

WAIST

HIPS

LEFT THIGH

RIGHT THIGH

LEFT CALF

RIGHT CALF

WEIGHT

NOTES

AFTER

DATE

CHEST

LEFT ARM

RIGHT ARM

WAIST

HIPS

LEFT THIGH

RIGHT THIGH

LEFT CALF

RIGHT CALF

WEIGHT

BODY MEASUREMENTS TRACKER

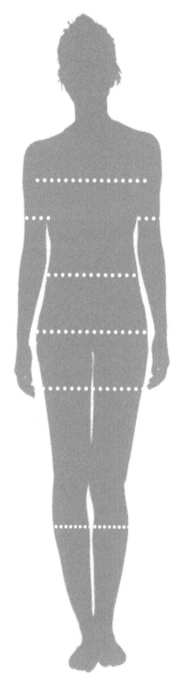

BEFORE

DATE

CHEST

LEFT ARM

RIGHT ARM

WAIST

HIPS

LEFT THIGH

RIGHT THIGH

LEFT CALF

RIGHT CALF

WEIGHT

NOTES

AFTER

DATE

CHEST

LEFT ARM

RIGHT ARM

WAIST

HIPS

LEFT THIGH

RIGHT THIGH

LEFT CALF

RIGHT CALF

WEIGHT

BODY MEASUREMENTS TRACKER

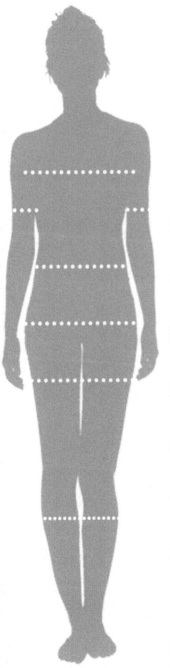

BEFORE

DATE

CHEST

LEFT ARM

RIGHT ARM

WAIST

HIPS

LEFT THIGH

RIGHT THIGH

LEFT CALF

RIGHT CALF

WEIGHT

NOTES

AFTER

DATE

CHEST

LEFT ARM

RIGHT ARM

WAIST

HIPS

LEFT THIGH

RIGHT THIGH

LEFT CALF

RIGHT CALF

WEIGHT

BODY MEASUREMENTS TRACKER

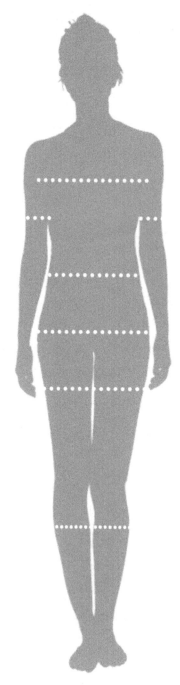

BEFORE

DATE

CHEST

LEFT ARM

RIGHT ARM

WAIST

HIPS

LEFT THIGH

RIGHT THIGH

LEFT CALF

RIGHT CALF

WEIGHT

NOTES

AFTER

DATE

CHEST

LEFT ARM

RIGHT ARM

WAIST

HIPS

LEFT THIGH

RIGHT THIGH

LEFT CALF

RIGHT CALF

WEIGHT

BODY MEASUREMENTS TRACKER

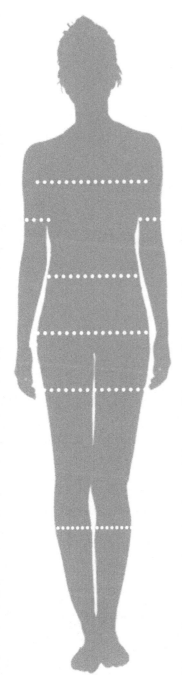

BEFORE

DATE

CHEST

LEFT ARM

RIGHT ARM

WAIST

HIPS

LEFT THIGH

RIGHT THIGH

LEFT CALF

RIGHT CALF

WEIGHT

NOTES

AFTER

DATE

CHEST

LEFT ARM

RIGHT ARM

WAIST

HIPS

LEFT THIGH

RIGHT THIGH

LEFT CALF

RIGHT CALF

WEIGHT

BODY MEASUREMENTS TRACKER

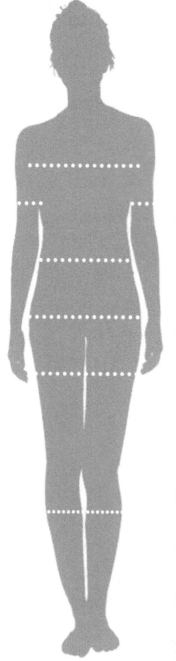

	BEFORE	AFTER
DATE		DATE
CHEST		CHEST
LEFT ARM		LEFT ARM
RIGHT ARM		RIGHT ARM
WAIST		WAIST
HIPS		HIPS
LEFT THIGH		LEFT THIGH
RIGHT THIGH		RIGHT THIGH
LEFT CALF		LEFT CALF
RIGHT CALF		RIGHT CALF
WEIGHT		WEIGHT
NOTES		

BODY MEASUREMENTS TRACKER

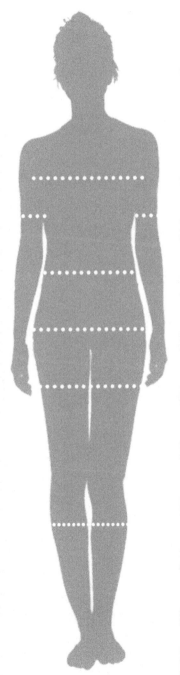

BEFORE

DATE

CHEST

LEFT ARM

RIGHT ARM

WAIST

HIPS

LEFT THIGH

RIGHT THIGH

LEFT CALF

RIGHT CALF

WEIGHT

NOTES

AFTER

DATE

CHEST

LEFT ARM

RIGHT ARM

WAIST

HIPS

LEFT THIGH

RIGHT THIGH

LEFT CALF

RIGHT CALF

WEIGHT

BODY MEASUREMENTS TRACKER

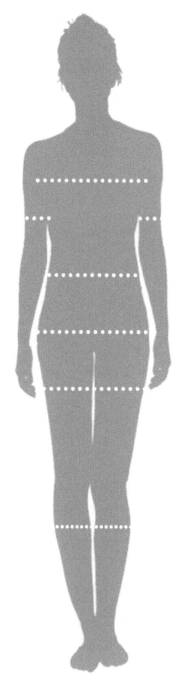

BEFORE

DATE

CHEST

LEFT ARM

RIGHT ARM

WAIST

HIPS

LEFT THIGH

RIGHT THIGH

LEFT CALF

RIGHT CALF

WEIGHT

NOTES

AFTER

DATE

CHEST

LEFT ARM

RIGHT ARM

WAIST

HIPS

LEFT THIGH

RIGHT THIGH

LEFT CALF

RIGHT CALF

WEIGHT

BODY MEASUREMENTS TRACKER

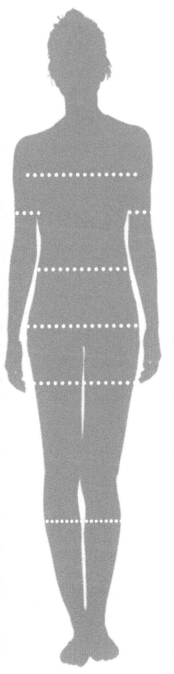

BEFORE

DATE

CHEST

LEFT ARM

RIGHT ARM

WAIST

HIPS

LEFT THIGH

RIGHT THIGH

LEFT CALF

RIGHT CALF

WEIGHT

NOTES

AFTER

DATE

CHEST

LEFT ARM

RIGHT ARM

WAIST

HIPS

LEFT THIGH

RIGHT THIGH

LEFT CALF

RIGHT CALF

WEIGHT

BODY MEASUREMENTS TRACKER

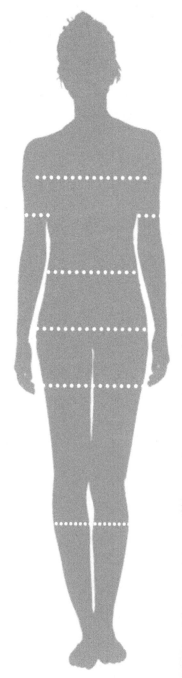

BEFORE

DATE

CHEST

LEFT ARM

RIGHT ARM

WAIST

HIPS

LEFT THIGH

RIGHT THIGH

LEFT CALF

RIGHT CALF

WEIGHT

NOTES

AFTER

DATE

CHEST

LEFT ARM

RIGHT ARM

WAIST

HIPS

LEFT THIGH

RIGHT THIGH

LEFT CALF

RIGHT CALF

WEIGHT

BODY MEASUREMENTS TRACKER

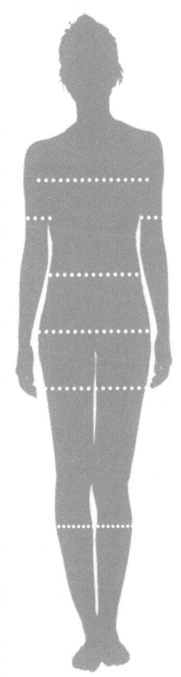

BEFORE

DATE

CHEST

LEFT ARM

RIGHT ARM

WAIST

HIPS

LEFT THIGH

RIGHT THIGH

LEFT CALF

RIGHT CALF

WEIGHT

NOTES

AFTER

DATE

CHEST

LEFT ARM

RIGHT ARM

WAIST

HIPS

LEFT THIGH

RIGHT THIGH

LEFT CALF

RIGHT CALF

WEIGHT

BODY MEASUREMENTS TRACKER

BEFORE   ## AFTER

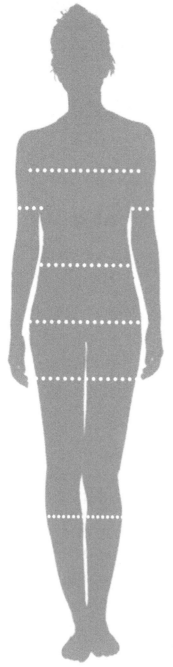

BEFORE	AFTER
DATE	DATE
CHEST	CHEST
LEFT ARM	LEFT ARM
RIGHT ARM	RIGHT ARM
WAIST	WAIST
HIPS	HIPS
LEFT THIGH	LEFT THIGH
RIGHT THIGH	RIGHT THIGH
LEFT CALF	LEFT CALF
RIGHT CALF	RIGHT CALF
WEIGHT	WEIGHT
NOTES	

BODY MEASUREMENTS TRACKER

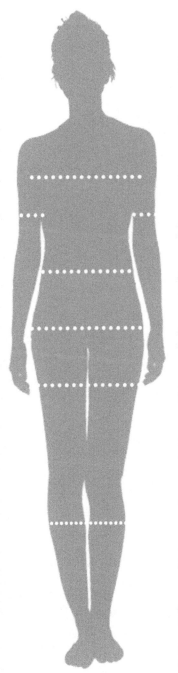

BEFORE

DATE

CHEST

LEFT ARM

RIGHT ARM

WAIST

HIPS

LEFT THIGH

RIGHT THIGH

LEFT CALF

RIGHT CALF

WEIGHT

NOTES

AFTER

DATE

CHEST

LEFT ARM

RIGHT ARM

WAIST

HIPS

LEFT THIGH

RIGHT THIGH

LEFT CALF

RIGHT CALF

WEIGHT

BODY MEASUREMENTS TRACKER

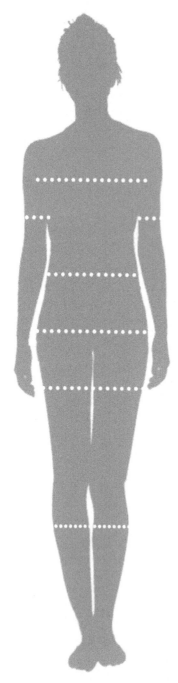

	BEFORE	AFTER
DATE		DATE
CHEST		CHEST
LEFT ARM		LEFT ARM
RIGHT ARM		RIGHT ARM
WAIST		WAIST
HIPS		HIPS
LEFT THIGH		LEFT THIGH
RIGHT THIGH		RIGHT THIGH
LEFT CALF		LEFT CALF
RIGHT CALF		RIGHT CALF
WEIGHT		WEIGHT
NOTES		

BODY MEASUREMENTS TRACKER

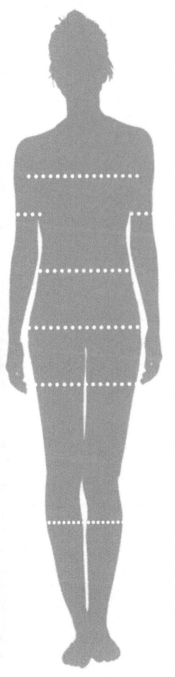

BEFORE

DATE

CHEST

LEFT ARM

RIGHT ARM

WAIST

HIPS

LEFT THIGH

RIGHT THIGH

LEFT CALF

RIGHT CALF

WEIGHT

NOTES

AFTER

DATE

CHEST

LEFT ARM

RIGHT ARM

WAIST

HIPS

LEFT THIGH

RIGHT THIGH

LEFT CALF

RIGHT CALF

WEIGHT

BODY MEASUREMENTS TRACKER

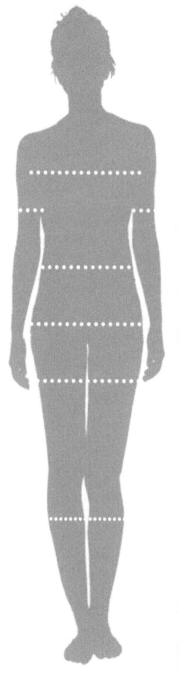

BEFORE

DATE

CHEST

LEFT ARM

RIGHT ARM

WAIST

HIPS

LEFT THIGH

RIGHT THIGH

LEFT CALF

RIGHT CALF

WEIGHT

NOTES

AFTER

DATE

CHEST

LEFT ARM

RIGHT ARM

WAIST

HIPS

LEFT THIGH

RIGHT THIGH

LEFT CALF

RIGHT CALF

WEIGHT

BODY MEASUREMENTS TRACKER

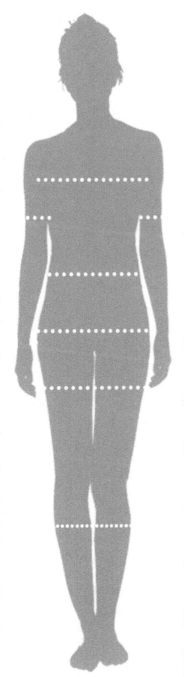

BEFORE

DATE

CHEST

LEFT ARM

RIGHT ARM

WAIST

HIPS

LEFT THIGH

RIGHT THIGH

LEFT CALF

RIGHT CALF

WEIGHT

NOTES

AFTER

DATE

CHEST

LEFT ARM

RIGHT ARM

WAIST

HIPS

LEFT THIGH

RIGHT THIGH

LEFT CALF

RIGHT CALF

WEIGHT

BODY MEASUREMENTS TRACKER

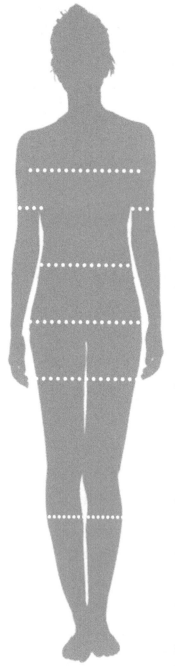

BEFORE

DATE

CHEST

LEFT ARM

RIGHT ARM

WAIST

HIPS

LEFT THIGH

RIGHT THIGH

LEFT CALF

RIGHT CALF

WEIGHT

NOTES

AFTER

DATE

CHEST

LEFT ARM

RIGHT ARM

WAIST

HIPS

LEFT THIGH

RIGHT THIGH

LEFI CALF

RIGHT CALF

WEIGHT

BODY MEASUREMENTS TRACKER

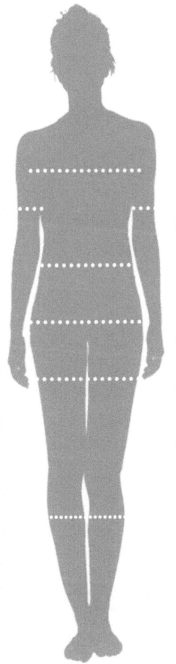

BEFORE

DATE

CHEST

LEFT ARM

RIGHT ARM

WAIST

HIPS

LEFT THIGH

RIGHT THIGH

LEFT CALF

RIGHT CALF

WEIGHT

NOTES

AFTER

DATE

CHEST

LEFT ARM

RIGHT ARM

WAIST

HIPS

LEFT THIGH

RIGHT THIGH

LEFT CALF

RIGHT CALF

WEIGHT

BODY MEASUREMENTS TRACKER

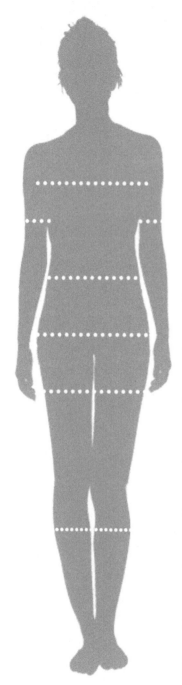

BEFORE

DATE

CHEST

LEFT ARM

RIGHT ARM

WAIST

HIPS

LEFT THIGH

RIGHT THIGH

LEFT CALF

RIGHT CALF

WEIGHT

NOTES

AFTER

DATE

CHEST

LEFT ARM

RIGHT ARM

WAIST

HIPS

LEFT THIGH

RIGHT THIGH

LEFT CALF

RIGHT CALF

WEIGHT

BODY MEASUREMENTS TRACKER

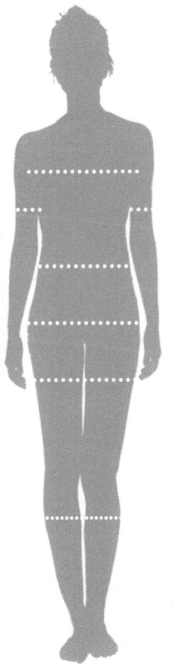

BEFORE

DATE

CHEST

LEFT ARM

RIGHT ARM

WAIST

HIPS

LEFT THIGH

RIGHT THIGH

LEFT CALF

RIGHT CALF

WEIGHT

NOTES

AFTER

DATE

CHEST

LEFT ARM

RIGHT ARM

WAIST

HIPS

LEFT THIGH

RIGHT THIGH

LEFT CALF

RIGHT CALF

WEIGHT

BODY MEASUREMENTS TRACKER

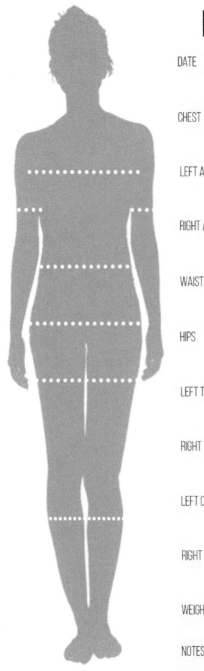

	BEFORE	AFTER
DATE		
CHEST		
LEFT ARM		
RIGHT ARM		
WAIST		
HIPS		
LEFT THIGH		
RIGHT THIGH		
LEFT CALF		
RIGHT CALF		
WEIGHT		
NOTES		

BODY MEASUREMENTS TRACKER

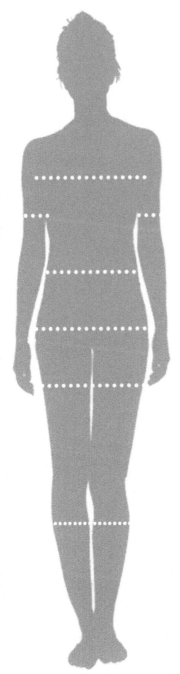

BEFORE

DATE

CHEST

LEFT ARM

RIGHT ARM

WAIST

HIPS

LEFT THIGH

RIGHT THIGH

LEFT CALF

RIGHT CALF

WEIGHT

NOTES

AFTER

DATE

CHEST

LEFT ARM

RIGHT ARM

WAIST

HIPS

LEFT THIGH

RIGHT THIGH

LEFT CALF

RIGHT CALF

WEIGHT

BODY MEASUREMENTS TRACKER

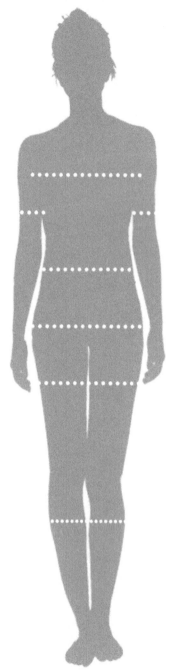

BEFORE

DATE

CHEST

LEFT ARM

RIGHT ARM

WAIST

HIPS

LEFT THIGH

RIGHT THIGH

LEFT CALF

RIGHT CALF

WEIGHT

NOTES

AFTER

DATE

CHEST

LEFT ARM

RIGHT ARM

WAIST

HIPS

LEFT THIGH

RIGHT THIGH

LEFT CALF

RIGHT CALF

WEIGHT

BODY MEASUREMENTS TRACKER

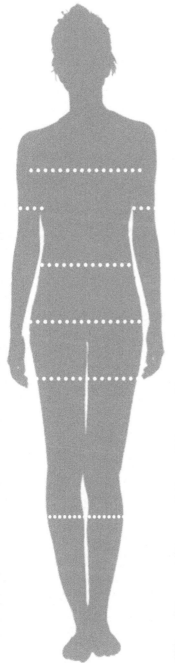

	BEFORE	AFTER
DATE		
CHEST		
LEFT ARM		
RIGHT ARM		
WAIST		
HIPS		
LEFT THIGH		
RIGHT THIGH		
LEFT CALF		
RIGHT CALF		
WEIGHT		
NOTES		

BODY MEASUREMENTS TRACKER

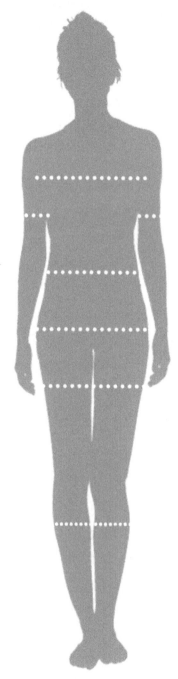

	BEFORE	AFTER
DATE		
CHEST		
LEFT ARM		
RIGHT ARM		
WAIST		
HIPS		
LEFT THIGH		
RIGHT THIGH		
LEFT CALF		
RIGHT CALF		
WEIGHT		
NOTES		

BODY MEASUREMENTS TRACKER

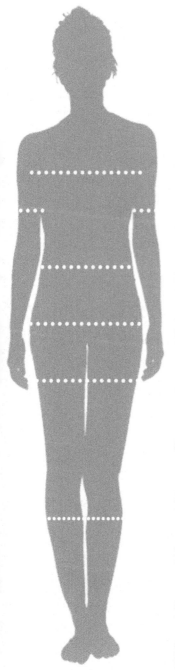

	BEFORE	AFTER
DATE		
CHEST		
LEFT ARM		
RIGHT ARM		
WAIST		
HIPS		
LEFT THIGH		
RIGHT THIGH		
LEFT CALF		
RIGHT CALF		
WEIGHT		
NOTES		

BODY MEASUREMENTS TRACKER

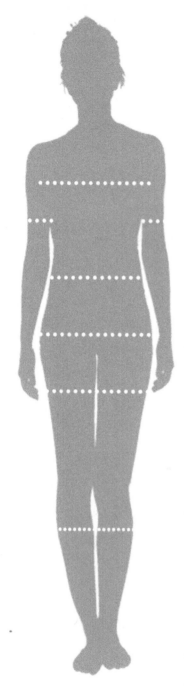

BEFORE

DATE

CHEST

LEFT ARM

RIGHT ARM

WAIST

HIPS

LEFT THIGH

RIGHT THIGH

LEFT CALF

RIGHT CALF

WEIGHT

NOTES

AFTER

DATE

CHEST

LEFT ARM

RIGHT ARM

WAIST

HIPS

LEFT THIGH

RIGHT THIGH

LEFT CALF

RIGHT CALF

WEIGHT

BODY MEASUREMENTS TRACKER

BEFORE

AFTER

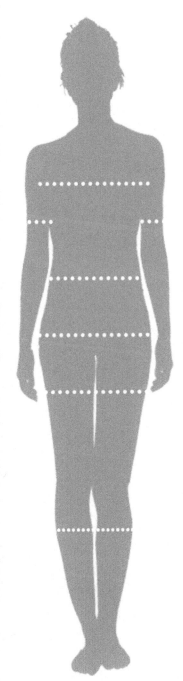

BEFORE	AFTER
DATE	DATE
CHEST	CHEST
LEFT ARM	LEFT ARM
RIGHT ARM	RIGHT ARM
WAIST	WAIST
HIPS	HIPS
LEFT THIGH	LEFT THIGH
RIGHT THIGH	RIGHT THIGH
LEFT CALF	LEFT CALF
RIGHT CALF	RIGHT CALF
WEIGHT	WEIGHT
NOTES	

BODY MEASUREMENTS TRACKER

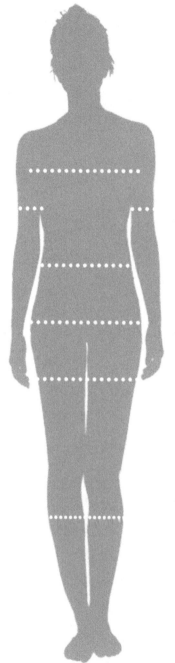

	BEFORE	AFTER
DATE		
CHEST		
LEFT ARM		
RIGHT ARM		
WAIST		
HIPS		
LEFT THIGH		
RIGHT THIGH		
LEFT CALF		
RIGHT CALF		
WEIGHT		
NOTES		

BODY MEASUREMENTS TRACKER

BEFORE

AFTER

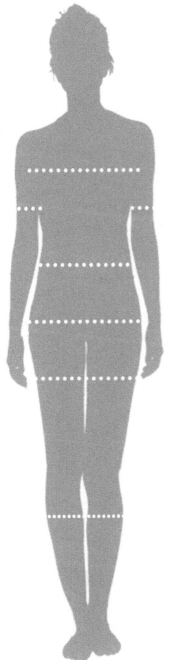

BEFORE	AFTER
DATE	DATE
CHEST	CHEST
LEFT ARM	LEFT ARM
RIGHT ARM	RIGHT ARM
WAIST	WAIST
HIPS	HIPS
LEFT THIGH	LEFT THIGH
RIGHT THIGH	RIGHT THIGH
LEFT CALF	LEFT CALF
RIGHT CALF	RIGHT CALF
WEIGHT	WEIGHT
NOTES	

BODY MEASUREMENTS TRACKER

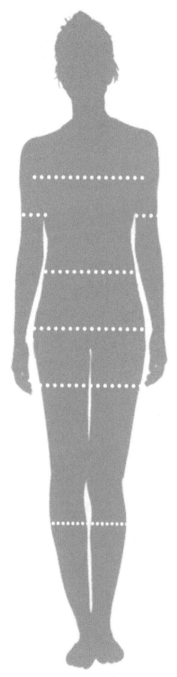

BEFORE

DATE

CHEST

LEFT ARM

RIGHT ARM

WAIST

HIPS

LEFT THIGH

RIGHT THIGH

LEFT CALF

RIGHT CALF

WEIGHT

NOTES

AFTER

DATE

CHEST

LEFT ARM

RIGHT ARM

WAIST

HIPS

LEFT THIGH

RIGHT THIGH

LEFT CALF

RIGHT CALF

WEIGHT

BODY MEASUREMENTS TRACKER

BEFORE

AFTER

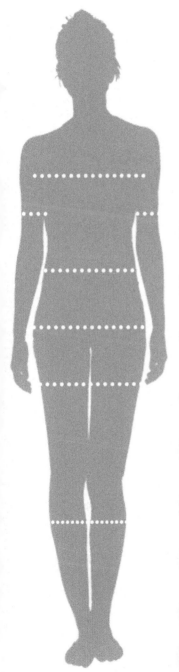

BEFORE	AFTER
DATE	DATE
CHEST	CHEST
LEFT ARM	LEFT ARM
RIGHT ARM	RIGHT ARM
WAIST	WAIST
HIPS	HIPS
LEFT THIGH	LEFT THIGH
RIGHT THIGH	RIGHT THIGH
LEFT CALF	LEFT CALF
RIGHT CALF	RIGHT CALF
WEIGHT	WEIGHT
NOTES	

BODY MEASUREMENTS TRACKER

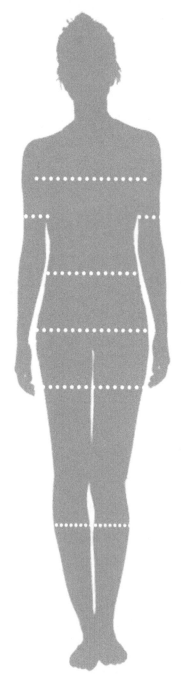

BEFORE

DATE

CHEST

LEFT ARM

RIGHT ARM

WAIST

HIPS

LEFT THIGH

RIGHT THIGH

LEFT CALF

RIGHT CALF

WEIGHT

NOTES

AFTER

DATE

CHEST

LEFT ARM

RIGHT ARM

WAIST

HIPS

LEFT THIGH

RIGHT THIGH

LEFT CALF

RIGHT CALF

WEIGHT

Made in the USA
Las Vegas, NV
02 May 2021